I0704071

MEDICINAL HERBS FOR MENTAL WELLNESS:
A GUIDE EXPLORING THE NEUROHERBAL INTERACTION

Medicinal Herbs for Mental Wellness:

A Guide Exploring the Neuroherbal Interaction

By

Tomas Dūminis

Copyright Statement

All rights reserved. No part of this book, "Medicinal Herbs for Mental Wellness: A Guide Exploring the Neuroherbal Interaction" may be reproduced, stored, or transmitted in any form or by any means, electronic, mechanical, photocopying, recording, scanning, or otherwise, without the prior written permission of the publisher, except for brief quotations embodied in critical reviews and certain other non-commercial uses permitted by copyright law.

Medicinal Herbs for Mental Wellness: a Guide Exploring the Neuroherbal Interaction 1st Edition.

ISBN: 9798322475910
Imprint: Independently published

Copyright © 2024 Tomas Dūminis

Disclaimer

This book is provided for educational purposes only and is not intended to serve as medical advice. The information contained herein is based on general knowledge and research and should not be used as a substitute for professional medical advice, diagnosis, or treatment. Readers are encouraged to consult with qualified healthcare professionals regarding any questions or concerns they may have regarding their health or medical conditions. The author and publisher do not accept any responsibility for any loss, injury, or damage incurred as a result of the use or reliance on the information provided in this book.

1 CONTENTS

2 INTRODUCTION

2.1 UNDERSTANDING ANXIETY

Anxiety is a common and normal human emotion characterized by feelings of worry, nervousness, or fear about future events, situations, or uncertainties. While it is natural to experience occasional anxiety in response to stressors or challenges, it becomes problematic when it is persistent, overwhelming, or interferes with daily functioning.

This complex emotion manifests differently in each individual, ranging from mild unease to severe panic. It can be triggered by a variety of factors, including personal relationships, work or school pressures, financial concerns, health issues, or traumatic experiences.

Understanding anxiety involves recognizing its various forms, such as generalized anxiety disorder (GAD), social anxiety disorder, panic disorder, phobias, and post-traumatic stress disorder (PTSD). Each of these conditions presents its own set of symptoms, which may include restlessness, irritability, difficulty concentrating, muscle tension, rapid heartbeat, sweating, trembling, and sleep disturbances.

Furthermore, anxiety often coexists with other mental health conditions, such as depression, making diagnosis and treatment more challenging. Despite its prevalence and impact, anxiety disorders are highly treatable through a combination of therapy, medication, lifestyle changes, and self-care strategies.

2.2 UNDERSTANDING STRESS

Stress is an inevitable part of the human experience, affecting individuals in myriad ways across all aspects of life. Defined as the body's response to any demand or challenge, stress can arise from both positive and negative situations, ranging from everyday hassles to major life changes. While some level of stress is normal and even beneficial, chronic, or excessive stress can have detrimental effects on physical, mental, and emotional well-being.

Understanding stress involves recognizing its multifaceted nature and the intricate interplay between external stressors and internal responses. External stressors may include work pressures, financial difficulties, relationship conflicts, academic demands, or environmental factors, while internal responses encompass physiological, cognitive, and emotional reactions.

Physiologically, stress triggers the body's "fight or flight" response, releasing hormones such as adrenaline and cortisol to prepare for action. This response can lead to heightened alertness, increased heart rate, rapid breathing, and tense muscles, which are adaptive in the short term but detrimental when prolonged.

Cognitively, stress can affect thinking patterns, leading to difficulty concentrating, memory problems, and negative thought patterns such as catastrophizing or rumination. Emotionally, stress often manifests as feelings of anxiety, frustration, anger, or sadness, further complicating one's ability to cope effectively.

Moreover, the impact of stress extends beyond the individual, influencing interpersonal relationships, work performance, and overall quality of life. Chronic stress has been linked to a myriad of health problems, including cardiovascular disease, digestive disorders, weakened immune function, and mental health conditions such as anxiety and depression.

Despite its ubiquity and potential negative consequences, stress management techniques and coping strategies can empower individuals to mitigate its effects and build resilience. Through self-care practices, mindfulness techniques, effective time management, social support, and seeking professional help when needed, individuals can navigate life's challenges with greater ease and adaptability.

2.3 UNDERSTANDING CAUSE AND EFFECT RELATIONSHIP

The intricate workings of the human brain have long fascinated scientists and scholars, particularly in understanding the complex interplay of neurotransmitters and their profound impact on mental wellbeing. Neurotransmitters are chemical messengers that facilitate communication between neurons, forming the foundation of brain function and behavior. The delicate balance of these neurotransmitters plays a pivotal role in regulating mood, cognition, emotion, and overall mental health.

At the forefront of this neurochemical orchestra are neurotransmitters such as serotonin, dopamine, norepinephrine, and gamma-aminobutyric acid (GABA), each with its unique functions and effects. Serotonin, often dubbed the "feel-good" neurotransmitter, is involved in regulating mood, sleep, appetite, and social behavior. Dopamine, known as the "reward" neurotransmitter, influences motivation, pleasure, and reinforcement learning. Norepinephrine contributes to arousal, attention, and stress response, while GABA acts as a calming agent, inhibiting neuronal activity and promoting relaxation.

The intricate balance of these neurotransmitters is crucial for maintaining optimal mental wellbeing. Dysregulation or imbalance of neurotransmitter levels has been implicated in various mental health disorders, including depression, anxiety, bipolar disorder, schizophrenia, and addiction. For instance, low levels of serotonin are associated with depressive symptoms, while disruptions in dopamine signaling have been linked to conditions like Parkinson's disease and addiction.

Understanding the role of neurotransmitters in mental health not only sheds light on the underlying mechanisms of psychiatric disorders but also informs treatment strategies. Psychotropic medications, such as selective serotonin reuptake inhibitors (SSRIs), serotonin-norepinephrine reuptake inhibitors (SNRIs), and antipsychotics, target specific neurotransmitter systems to alleviate symptoms and restore balance. Additionally, psychotherapy, lifestyle modifications, and holistic approaches can complement pharmacological interventions in promoting mental wellness. Moreover, emerging research highlights the influence of environmental factors, genetics, epigenetics, and neuroplasticity on neurotransmitter function and mental health outcomes. This interdisciplinary approach underscores the complexity of mental wellbeing and the need for personalized, comprehensive interventions.

In this exploration of neurotransmitters and mental wellbeing, we delve into their intricate mechanisms, roles in psychiatric disorders, and implications for treatment and prevention. By resolving the mysteries of the brain's chemical messengers, we strive to advance our understanding of mental health and enhance strategies for promoting resilience, recovery, and flourishing in individuals and communities alike.

2.4 FUNDAMENTALS OF NEUROSCIENCE

The nervous system is a complex network of specialized cells and tissues that coordinates and regulates the functions of the body. From basic reflexes to complex thoughts and behaviors, the nervous system plays a crucial

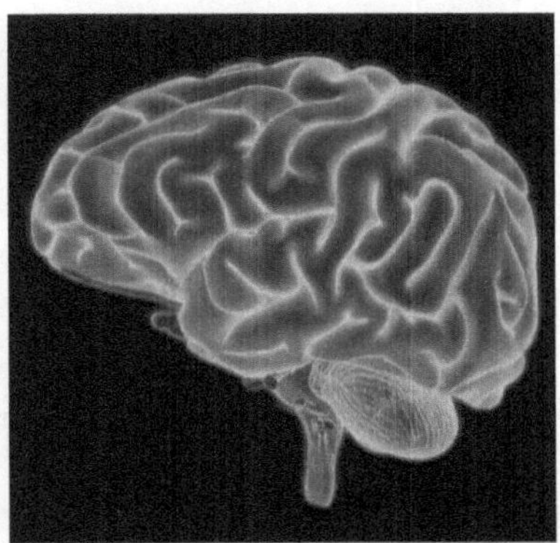

role in every aspect of human experience. In this chapter, we will explore the structure and function of the nervous system, from the basic building blocks of neurons to the intricate networks that enable communication and control throughout the body.

2.4.1 Structure of the Nervous System

The nervous system is divided into two main components: the central nervous system (CNS) and the peripheral nervous system (PNS). The CNS consists of the brain and spinal cord, while the PNS includes all the nerves that extend from the CNS to the rest of the body. The brain is the command center of the nervous system, responsible for processing sensory information, coordinating motor responses, and regulating higher cognitive functions. The spinal cord serves as a relay station, transmitting signals between the brain and the body and coordinating reflex responses.

2.4.2   Neurotransmission

Neurons are the fundamental units of the nervous system, responsible for transmitting electrical and chemical signals throughout the body. Each neuron consists of a cell body, dendrites, and an axon. Dendrites receive incoming signals from other neurons, while the axon transmits signals away from the cell body to other neurons or target cells. Neurons communicate with each other through specialized junctions called synapses, where neurotransmitters are released from the axon terminals of one neuron and bind to receptors on the dendrites of another neuron.

2.4.3   Electrical Signaling

The transmission of signals within neurons is primarily electrical in nature, driven by changes in membrane potential. Neurons maintain a resting membrane potential, with a negative charge inside the cell relative to the outside. When a neuron is stimulated, ion channels in the cell membrane open, allowing ions such as sodium and potassium to flow in and out of the cell, altering the membrane potential and generating an electrical signal known as an action potential. Action potentials propagate along the length of the axon, enabling rapid communication between neurons.

2.4.4   Chemical Signaling

At synapses, communication between neurons occurs through chemical signaling mediated by neurotransmitters. Neurotransmitters are released from the presynaptic neuron in response to an action potential and diffuse across the synaptic cleft to bind to receptors on the postsynaptic neuron, triggering a response. Excitatory neurotransmitters such as glutamate depolarize the postsynaptic membrane, increasing the likelihood of an action potential, while inhibitory neurotransmitters such as GABA hyperpolarize the membrane, decreasing neuronal activity.

2.4.5   Integration and Processing

The nervous system integrates and processes incoming sensory information, coordinating appropriate responses to internal and external stimuli. Sensory neurons transmit signals from sensory receptors to the CNS, where the information is processed and interpreted by interneurons in the brain and spinal cord. Motor neurons then transmit signals from the CNS to muscles and glands, coordinating motor responses. Through a complex network of interconnected neurons and neural circuits, the nervous system regulates physiological functions, behaviors, and emotions.

The nervous system is a remarkable biological system that enables communication and coordination throughout the body. From the basic mechanisms of neuronal signaling to the intricate networks of the brain, the nervous system governs every aspect of human experience, from sensation and movement to cognition and emotion. By understanding how the nervous system works, we can gain insight into the mechanisms underlying normal function and dysfunction, paving the way for new approaches to treating neurological disorders and enhancing human health and well-being.

2.5 HELPING THE NERVOUS SYSTEM TO STAY HEALTHY

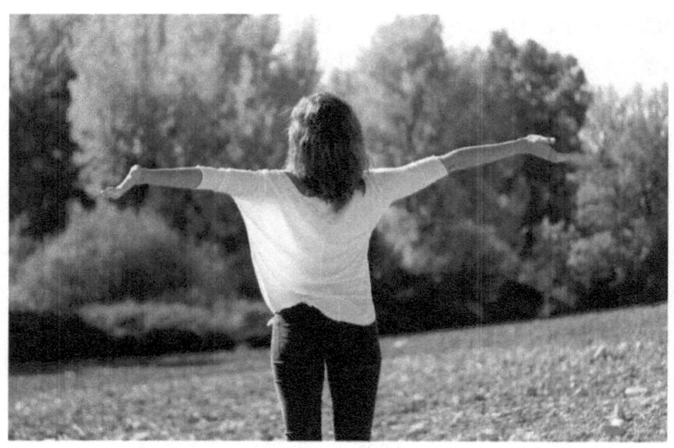

Helping the nervous system naturally involves a holistic approach that encompasses lifestyle modifications, dietary adjustments, and the incorporation of specific nutrients and herbs into one's routine. Firstly, maintaining a balanced diet is paramount, as it provides essential nutrients crucial for supporting nervous system health. A diet rich in antioxidants, vitamins (especially B vitamins), and minerals like magnesium and zinc supports nerve function and neurotransmitter synthesis. Additionally, including sources of omega-3 fatty acids, such as fatty fish, flaxseeds, and walnuts, can offer anti-inflammatory properties and aid in maintaining neuronal structure and function.

Herbal remedies have long been utilized to support nervous system health and alleviate symptoms of stress and anxiety. Chamomile, Valerian, Lavender, Lemon Balm, and Passionflower are among the herbs known for their calming and mood-enhancing effects. These herbs can be consumed in various forms, including teas, tinctures, or supplements.

Mind-body practices, including mindfulness meditation, yoga, tai chi, and qigong, offer effective ways to reduce stress, enhance relaxation, and improve overall well-being. These practices regulate the autonomic nervous system, boost mood, and build resilience to stressors.

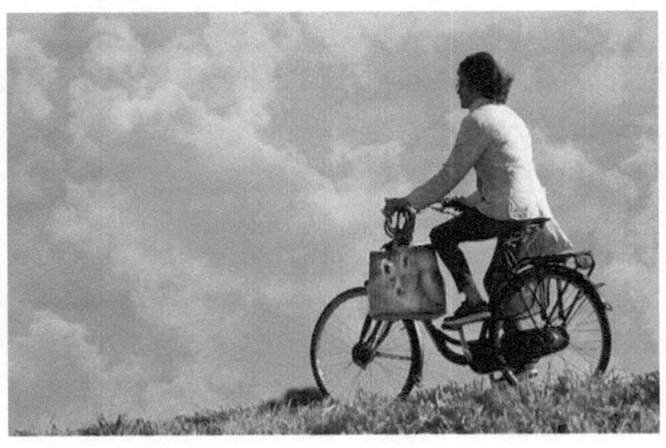

Regular physical activity is essential for supporting nervous system health, as it improves mood, reduces stress, and enhances cognitive function. Combining aerobic exercise like walking or jogging with strength training supports overall nervous system health. Stress reduction techniques, such as deep breathing exercises, progressive muscle relaxation, and guided imagery, can effectively promote relaxation and alleviate stress. Adequate sleep is crucial for nervous system function and overall health, so establishing a consistent sleep schedule and creating a relaxing bedtime routine is essential.

Limiting alcohol consumption and reducing caffeine intake can also support nervous system health by avoiding disruptions in nervous system function and sleep patterns. Staying hydrated throughout the day is important, as dehydration can impair cognitive function and mood. Drinking plenty of water and consuming hydrating foods like fruits and vegetables supports nervous system hydration. Lastly, seeking guidance from a healthcare professional is advisable if experiencing persistent or severe symptoms related to nervous system health. They can offer personalized recommendations and develop a comprehensive plan to support nervous system function and overall well-being.

3 NEUROTRANSMITTERS RELATED TO MOOD

Now that we have established the function and importance of the natural "chemical" messengers in the brain, let's dive a little deeper into understanding their structure and function.

3.1 ACETYLCHOLINE

Acetylcholine (ACh) stands as one of the most fundamental neurotransmitters in the human body, playing a pivotal role in the intricate network of communication within the nervous system. First discovered in the early 20th century, acetylcholine has since been extensively studied for its diverse functions in both the central and peripheral nervous systems.

At its core, acetylcholine serves as a key mediator of neuronal signaling, facilitating the transmission of nerve impulses across synapses. Understanding the structure and function of acetylcholine unveils its profound impact on various physiological processes, ranging from muscle contraction and cognition to autonomic nervous system regulation.

Structurally, acetylcholine is a simple molecule composed of an acetyl group attached to a choline molecule. This neurotransmitter is synthesized within nerve terminals by the enzyme choline acetyltransferase, utilizing acetyl coenzyme A (acetyl-CoA) and choline as precursor molecules. Once synthesized, acetylcholine is stored in synaptic vesicles, awaiting release in response to neuronal stimulation.

Functionally, acetylcholine exerts its effects through interactions with two classes of receptors: nicotinic acetylcholine receptors (nAChRs) and muscarinic acetylcholine receptors (mAChRs). Nicotinic receptors are ligand-gated ion channels found in the central and peripheral nervous systems, mediating fast excitatory neurotransmission at neuromuscular junctions and within certain brain regions. Muscarinic receptors, on the other hand, are G protein-coupled receptors distributed throughout the central and peripheral nervous systems, regulating a wide array of physiological functions, including heart rate, smooth muscle contraction, glandular secretion, and neurotransmitter release.

The multifaceted roles of acetylcholine extend beyond its involvement in neurotransmission. In the peripheral nervous system, acetylcholine serves as the primary neurotransmitter at neuromuscular junctions, facilitating muscle contraction and movement. Within the autonomic nervous system, acetylcholine modulates both sympathetic and parasympathetic responses, exerting control over heart rate, gastrointestinal motility, and other visceral functions.

In the central nervous system, acetylcholine plays a crucial role in cognitive processes such as attention, learning, and memory. Dysfunction of cholinergic neurotransmission has been implicated in neurodegenerative disorders such as Alzheimer's disease, highlighting the significance of acetylcholine in maintaining cognitive function and brain health.

3.2 DOPAMINE

Dopamine, often referred to as the "reward" neurotransmitter, stands as a cornerstone of the brain's intricate communication system, exerting profound effects on a myriad of physiological processes and behaviors. Since its discovery in the mid-20th century, dopamine has captivated researchers and clinicians alike for its central role in modulating mood, motivation, movement, and cognitive function.

Structurally, dopamine is a monoamine neurotransmitter belonging to the catecholamine family, synthesized from the amino acid tyrosine through a series of enzymatic reactions. Within neurons, the enzyme tyrosine hydroxylase converts tyrosine into L-DOPA, which is then further metabolized into dopamine by the enzyme aromatic L-amino acid decarboxylase. This neurotransmitter is synthesized predominantly in dopaminergic neurons located in various brain regions, including the substantia nigra and the ventral tegmental area.

Functionally, dopamine exerts its effects through interactions with a diverse array of dopamine receptors, categorized into two main families: D1-like receptors (D1 and D5 subtypes) and D2-like receptors (D2, D3, and D4 subtypes). These receptors are distributed throughout the central nervous system, with distinct regional and cellular expression patterns, influencing a wide range of physiological and behavioral functions.

Dopamine's influence on the brain's reward circuitry is perhaps its most well-known function. In this context, dopamine plays a critical role in encoding pleasurable experiences, reinforcing behaviors that lead to reward, and motivating goal-directed actions. Dysfunction of the dopamine system has been implicated in addiction, as well as various neuropsychiatric disorders such as depression, schizophrenia, and Parkinson's disease.

Beyond its role in reward processing, dopamine is also crucial for motor control and coordination. In the basal ganglia, dopaminergic projections from the substantia nigra pars compacta modulate the initiation and execution of voluntary movements. Dysregulation of dopamine signaling in this circuitry underlies the motor symptoms observed in Parkinson's disease, a neurodegenerative disorder characterized by the loss of dopaminergic neurons.

Furthermore, dopamine plays a vital role in cognitive processes such as attention, working memory, and executive function. Alterations in dopaminergic neurotransmission have been implicated in attention deficit hyperactivity disorder (ADHD) and other cognitive disorders, highlighting the significance of dopamine in maintaining optimal cognitive function.

3.3 SEROTONIN

Serotonin, often dubbed the "molecule of happiness," is a neurotransmitter that holds a prominent role in regulating a wide array of physiological processes and behaviors within the human body. Since its discovery in the mid-20th century, serotonin has captivated researchers and clinicians for its profound influence on mood, emotion, cognition, sleep, appetite, and various other functions.

Structurally, serotonin, also known as 5-hydroxytryptamine (5-HT), is a monoamine neurotransmitter synthesized from the amino acid tryptophan through a series of enzymatic reactions. Within neurons, tryptophan hydroxylase catalyzes the conversion of tryptophan into 5-hydroxytryptophan (5-HTP), which is then further metabolized into serotonin by the enzyme aromatic L-amino acid decarboxylase. Serotonin is primarily synthesized in serotonergic neurons located in clusters within the raphe nuclei of the brainstem.

Functionally, serotonin exerts its effects through interactions with a diverse array of serotonin receptors, classified into several families (5-HT1 to 5-HT7), each with multiple subtypes. These receptors are distributed throughout the central nervous system and peripheral tissues, with distinct regional and cellular expression patterns, influencing a myriad of physiological and behavioral functions.

One of serotonin's most well-known functions is its role in regulating mood and emotion. Serotonergic projections from the raphe nuclei innervate various brain regions implicated in emotional processing, including the amygdala, prefrontal cortex, and hippocampus. Serotonin is believed to play a crucial role in mood stabilization, stress response, and emotional regulation. Dysregulation of the serotonin system has been implicated in mood disorders such as depression and anxiety.

In addition to its effects on mood, serotonin also modulates appetite and satiety, contributing to the regulation of food intake and energy balance. Serotonergic signaling influences feeding behavior through its interactions with hypothalamic circuits involved in appetite regulation and reward processing. Dysfunction of the serotonin system has been linked to eating disorders such as anorexia nervosa and bulimia nervosa.

Furthermore, serotonin plays a critical role in sleep-wake regulation and circadian rhythms. Serotonergic neurons in the brainstem raphe nuclei contribute to the modulation of sleep stages and arousal states. Pharmacological agents that enhance serotonin signaling, such as selective serotonin reuptake inhibitors (SSRIs), are commonly used in the treatment of sleep disorders such as insomnia.

3.4 NOREPINEPHRINE

Norepinephrine, also known as noradrenaline, is a neurotransmitter that plays a vital role in the functioning of the human body, influencing a wide range of physiological processes and behaviors. Its intricate interplay within the central and peripheral nervous systems underscores its significance in regulating arousal, attention, mood, stress response, and autonomic functions.

Structurally, norepinephrine is a catecholamine neurotransmitter synthesized from the amino acid tyrosine through a series of enzymatic reactions. Within neurons, the enzyme tyrosine hydroxylase converts tyrosine into L-DOPA, which is then further metabolized into dopamine. Dopamine is subsequently converted into norepinephrine by the enzyme dopamine beta-hydroxylase, primarily within noradrenergic neurons located in the locus coeruleus of the brainstem.

Functionally, norepinephrine exerts its effects through interactions with adrenergic receptors, which are divided into two main classes: alpha-adrenergic receptors and beta-adrenergic receptors. These receptors are distributed throughout the central and peripheral nervous systems, with diverse regional and cellular expression patterns, influencing a myriad of physiological and behavioral functions.

One of norepinephrine's primary functions is its role in the regulation of arousal and attention. Noradrenergic projections from the locus coeruleus innervate various brain regions implicated in attentional processes, including the prefrontal cortex, thalamus, and hippocampus. Norepinephrine is believed to enhance vigilance, alertness, and cognitive performance, promoting adaptive responses to environmental stimuli.

In addition to its effects on arousal and attention, norepinephrine is also involved in the regulation of mood and emotional processing. Noradrenergic signaling influences emotional responses through its interactions with limbic structures such as the amygdala and the bed nucleus of the stria terminalis. Dysregulation of the noradrenergic system has been implicated in mood disorders such as depression and anxiety.

Furthermore, norepinephrine plays a critical role in the autonomic nervous system, regulating functions such as heart rate, blood pressure, and gastrointestinal motility. Noradrenergic neurons in the sympathetic nervous system release norepinephrine as a neurotransmitter, mediating the "fight or flight" response to stressors. Pharmacological agents that modulate noradrenergic signaling, such as alpha and beta blockers, are commonly used in the treatment of cardiovascular conditions and hypertension.

3.5 EPINEPHRINE

Epinephrine, also known as adrenaline, stands as a pivotal neurotransmitter and hormone in the human body, orchestrating an array of physiological responses crucial for survival in the face of stress and danger. Its intricate interplay within the neuroendocrine system underscores its significance in regulating the "fight or flight" response, as well as various other bodily functions.

Structurally, epinephrine is a catecholamine neurotransmitter synthesized from the amino acid tyrosine through a series of enzymatic reactions. Within neurons of the adrenal medulla, the enzyme tyrosine hydroxylase converts tyrosine into L-DOPA, which is then further metabolized into dopamine. Dopamine is subsequently converted into norepinephrine by the enzyme dopamine beta-hydroxylase, and finally into epinephrine by phenylethanolamine N-methyltransferase.

Functionally, epinephrine exerts its effects through interactions with adrenergic receptors, similar to norepinephrine. These receptors are classified into two main classes: alpha-adrenergic receptors and beta-adrenergic receptors, each with multiple subtypes. Adrenergic receptors are distributed throughout the body, influencing a myriad of physiological and behavioral responses.

One of epinephrine's primary functions is its role in the initiation and orchestration of the "fight or flight" response. In moments of stress or danger, the adrenal glands release epinephrine into the bloodstream, triggering a cascade of physiological changes designed to prepare the body for action. These changes include increased heart rate, dilation of airways, redirection of blood flow to vital organs, and mobilization of energy reserves. Collectively, these responses enhance physical performance and increase the likelihood of survival in threatening situations.

Beyond its role in the stress response, epinephrine also plays a critical role in regulating cardiovascular function. Epinephrine acts on beta-adrenergic receptors in the heart to increase cardiac output and elevate blood pressure, ensuring adequate perfusion of tissues during times of heightened demand. Additionally, epinephrine stimulates glycogenolysis and lipolysis in the liver and adipose tissue, releasing glucose and fatty acids into the bloodstream to provide fuel for energy-intensive activities.

Furthermore, epinephrine influences various other physiological processes, including metabolism, immune function, and neurotransmission. Its effects are diverse and widespread, reflecting its central role in coordinating adaptive responses to environmental challenges.

3.6 GAMMA-AMINOBUTYRIC ACID

Gamma-aminobutyric acid, or GABA, holds a unique and vital role within the intricate network of neurotransmitters in the human brain. As the principal inhibitory neurotransmitter, GABA exerts profound effects on neuronal signaling, modulating brain activity to maintain a delicate balance between excitation and inhibition. Its structural simplicity belies its complex functionality, making it a central focus of research in neuroscience and pharmacology.

Structurally, GABA is a non-protein amino acid synthesized from the neurotransmitter glutamate through the action of the enzyme glutamate decarboxylase. This conversion involves the removal of a carboxyl group from glutamate, resulting in the formation of GABA. Once synthesized, GABA is packaged into synaptic vesicles and released from presynaptic terminals in response to neuronal activity.

Functionally, GABA acts predominantly through its interaction with two classes of receptors: GABAA receptors and GABAB receptors. GABAA receptors are ligand-gated ion channels composed of multiple subunits, which, upon activation by GABA, allow the influx of chloride ions into the neuron, hyperpolarizing the cell membrane and inhibiting neuronal firing. GABAB receptors, on the other hand, are G protein-coupled receptors that modulate neurotransmitter release and cellular excitability through a cascade of intracellular signaling events.

The inhibitory effects of GABA play a crucial role in shaping neural circuits and regulating brain function. By counteracting the excitatory actions of neurotransmitters such as glutamate, GABA helps maintain neuronal stability and prevent runaway excitation that can lead to seizures or neuronal damage. Moreover, GABAergic neurotransmission is involved in various physiological processes, including sleep, anxiety, muscle tone, and motor coordination.

Dysfunction of the GABAergic system has been implicated in numerous neurological and psychiatric disorders. For example, reduced GABAergic activity has been observed in epilepsy, anxiety disorders, and sleep disorders, while excessive GABAergic inhibition is associated with conditions such as depression and schizophrenia. Pharmacological agents that enhance GABAergic neurotransmission, such as benzodiazepines and barbiturates, are commonly used in the treatment of anxiety, insomnia, and seizures.

3.7 GLUTAMATE

Glutamate, the most abundant excitatory neurotransmitter in the human brain, serves as a fundamental player in orchestrating neural communication and shaping brain function. Its multifaceted role extends beyond neurotransmission, encompassing critical functions in synaptic plasticity, learning, memory, and various physiological processes. The intricate interplay of glutamate within neural circuits underlies its significance as a key mediator of cognitive and behavioral processes.

Structurally, glutamate is a simple amino acid with a carboxylic acid side chain, synthesized from the precursor molecule α-ketoglutarate through a series of enzymatic reactions. Within neurons, glutamate is synthesized by the enzyme glutaminase from glutamine, or by the enzyme glutamate dehydrogenase from α-ketoglutarate. Once synthesized, glutamate is packaged into synaptic vesicles and released from presynaptic terminals in response to neuronal activity.

Functionally, glutamate exerts its effects through interactions with a diverse array of glutamate receptors, categorized into two main classes: ionotropic glutamate receptors and metabotropic glutamate receptors. Ionotropic receptors, including NMDA receptors, AMPA receptors, and kainate receptors, are ligand-gated ion channels that mediate fast excitatory neurotransmission. Metabotropic receptors, on the other hand, are G protein-coupled receptors that modulate neuronal excitability and synaptic transmission through intracellular signaling pathways.

The excitatory effects of glutamate play a central role in neuronal communication and synaptic plasticity. By activating postsynaptic glutamate receptors, glutamate promotes depolarization of the cell membrane and initiates action potentials, leading to the transmission of electrical signals between neurons. Moreover, glutamatergic neurotransmission is essential for synaptic plasticity mechanisms such as long-term potentiation (LTP) and long-term depression (LTD), which underlie learning and memory processes.

Beyond its role in neurotransmission and synaptic plasticity, glutamate is involved in various physiological processes throughout the body. Glutamatergic signaling influences motor function, sensory perception, hormonal regulation, and metabolic pathways, highlighting its widespread impact on organismal homeostasis and function.

Dysregulation of glutamatergic neurotransmission has been implicated in numerous neurological and psychiatric disorders. Excessive glutamate release and impaired glutamate clearance have been associated with excitotoxicity and neuronal damage in conditions such as stroke, traumatic brain injury, and neurodegenerative diseases like Alzheimer's and Parkinson's. Moreover, alterations in glutamatergic signaling have been linked to psychiatric disorders such as depression, schizophrenia, and addiction.

3.8 OXYTOCIN

Oxytocin, often referred to as the "love hormone" or "bonding hormone," plays a central role in social behavior, attachment, and reproductive physiology in humans and other mammals. This neuropeptide, produced in the hypothalamus and released by the pituitary gland, exerts a wide range of effects on both the brain and the body, influencing emotional responses, social interactions, and various physiological processes.

Structurally, oxytocin is a peptide composed of nine amino acids, making it relatively small in size compared to other neuropeptides. It is synthesized as part of a larger precursor molecule called oxytocin/neurophysin I, which is cleaved to release the active form of oxytocin. Upon release, oxytocin binds to specific receptors known as oxytocin receptors, which are distributed throughout the brain and peripheral tissues.

Functionally, oxytocin modulates a diverse array of physiological and behavioral processes, with its effects varying depending on the context and target tissue. In the brain, oxytocin influences social behavior by promoting bonding, trust, and empathy. It enhances social recognition, facilitates maternal-infant attachment, and fosters affiliative behaviors such as pair bonding and maternal care.

Oxytocin's role in reproductive physiology is perhaps its most well-known function. During childbirth, oxytocin promotes uterine contractions, facilitating labor and delivery. After birth, oxytocin stimulates milk ejection (let-down reflex) from the mammary glands, enabling breastfeeding and maternal care. These reproductive functions underscore oxytocin's importance in facilitating parent-infant bonding and nurturing behavior.

Beyond its effects on social behavior and reproduction, oxytocin also influences stress responses, pain perception, and cardiovascular function. Oxytocin has been shown to reduce levels of cortisol (the stress hormone) and modulate pain sensitivity, leading to its potential therapeutic applications in stress-related disorders and chronic pain management.

Dysregulation of oxytocin signaling has been implicated in various psychiatric disorders and social deficits. Reduced oxytocin levels or impaired oxytocin receptor function have been associated with conditions such as autism spectrum disorder, social anxiety disorder, and depression. Understanding the mechanisms underlying oxytocin's effects on brain function and behavior may offer insights into novel therapeutic approaches for these conditions.

3.9 ENDORPHINS

Endorphins, often referred to as the "feel-good" hormones, are a class of neurotransmitters and neuropeptides that play a crucial role in modulating pain perception, mood, and stress responses within the human body. These endogenous opioid peptides are produced in various regions of the brain and spinal cord, as well as in peripheral tissues, and exert powerful effects on both physical and emotional well-being.

Structurally, endorphins belong to the family of opioid peptides, which includes beta-endorphins, enkephalins, and dynorphins, among others. These peptides are composed of amino acids and are derived from larger precursor molecules that are cleaved to release the active forms of endorphins. Endorphins bind to and activate opioid receptors, which are distributed throughout the central nervous system and peripheral tissues, initiating a cascade of physiological responses.

Functionally, endorphins act as natural painkillers and mood enhancers, playing a critical role in the body's ability to cope with stress and discomfort. Upon activation of opioid receptors, endorphins inhibit the transmission of pain signals in the spinal cord and brain, resulting in analgesia and feelings of euphoria. This pain-relieving effect is particularly pronounced during strenuous physical activity, such as exercise, where endorphin release is believed to contribute to the phenomenon known as "runner's high."

In addition to their analgesic properties, endorphins also influence mood regulation and emotional well-being. Endorphin release is associated with feelings of pleasure, relaxation, and contentment, contributing to the sense of reward and satisfaction experienced during enjoyable activities. Moreover, endorphins play a role in modulating stress responses, helping to mitigate the physiological effects of acute and chronic stressors on the body.

Beyond their effects on pain perception and mood, endorphins have been implicated in various physiological processes, including immune function, gastrointestinal motility, and cardiovascular regulation. Endorphin release has been shown to modulate immune cell activity and inflammation, suggesting a potential role in immune-mediated disorders and inflammatory diseases.

Dysregulation of endorphin signaling has been implicated in conditions such as chronic pain, mood disorders, and addiction. Reduced endorphin levels or impaired endorphin receptor function may contribute to heightened pain sensitivity, dysphoria, and maladaptive coping strategies. Understanding the mechanisms underlying endorphin function and dysregulation may offer insights into novel therapeutic approaches for these conditions.

4 HERBAL INTERACTIONS WITH THE NERVOUS SYSTEM

The interactions between compounds found in herbs and nerve receptors is a fascinating area of study that bridges traditional herbal medicine and modern pharmacology. Across cultures and throughout history, humans have turned to plants for their therapeutic properties, recognizing their potential to influence various physiological processes, including those mediated by the nervous system. Understanding how these compounds interact with nerve receptors provides valuable insight into the mechanisms underlying herbal remedies and their effects on human health.

Herbs contain a myriad of bioactive compounds, including alkaloids, flavonoids, terpenes, and phenolic acids, among others, each with its unique chemical structure and biological activity. Many of these compounds have been found to interact with nerve receptors, modulating neurotransmission and influencing neural signaling pathways.

One common mode of interaction involves the binding of herbal compounds to specific receptors on the surface of neurons, mimicking or antagonizing the actions of endogenous neurotransmitters. For example, alkaloids such as morphine and nicotine found in opium poppy (*Papaver somniferum*) and tobacco (*Nicotiana tabacum*), respectively, exert their effects by binding to opioid receptors and nicotinic acetylcholine receptors in the central and peripheral nervous systems.

Moreover, herbal compounds may influence the activity of neurotransmitter transporters, enzymes, or ion channels involved in synaptic transmission and neuronal excitability. For instance, flavonoids present in Ginkgo biloba have been shown to inhibit the reuptake of serotonin and norepinephrine, thereby prolonging the action of these neurotransmitters and modulating mood and cognition.

Additionally, some herbal compounds possess neuroprotective properties, shielding neurons from damage caused by oxidative stress, inflammation, or excitotoxicity. Polyphenols found in green tea (*Camellia sinensis*), for example, have been shown to scavenge free radicals, attenuate neuroinflammation, and promote neuronal survival, potentially offering therapeutic benefits in neurodegenerative diseases like Alzheimer's and Parkinson's.

Furthermore, herbal compounds can influence intracellular signaling cascades and gene expression patterns within neurons, thereby regulating neuroplasticity, synaptic connectivity, and neuronal survival. Compounds such as curcumin from turmeric (*Curcuma longa*) and resveratrol from grapes (*Vitis vinifera*) have been found to modulate the activity of various kinases, transcription factors, and neurotrophic factors, promoting neuronal growth, differentiation, and synaptic remodeling.

Despite the wealth of knowledge amassed on the interactions between herbal compounds and nerve receptors, much remains to be explored. The complexity of herbal formulations, the variability in bioavailability and metabolism of phytochemicals, and the diverse array of nerve receptors present challenges in elucidating their mechanisms of action. Nonetheless, the integration of traditional herbal knowledge with modern scientific methods holds promise for uncovering novel therapeutic agents and optimizing herbal remedies for the promotion of brain health and the treatment of neurological and psychiatric disorders.

4.1 CHAMOMILE

Chamomile (*Matricaria chamomilla*) is a widely recognized medicinal herb known for its calming properties and therapeutic effects on the nervous system. For centuries,

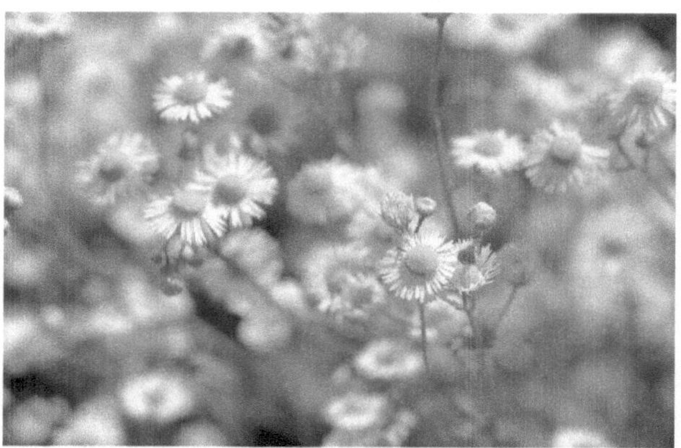

chamomile has been used in traditional medicine practices across cultures to alleviate anxiety, promote relaxation, and improve sleep quality. While its mechanisms of action are multifaceted and not fully understood, scientific research has begun to unravel the ways in which chamomile interacts with the nervous system, shedding light on its potential as a natural remedy for various neurological and psychological conditions.

Chamomile contains a diverse array of bioactive compounds, including flavonoids, terpenoids, and essential oils, which contribute to its pharmacological effects. Among these compounds, apigenin, bisabolol, and chamazulene have garnered particular attention for their ability to modulate neural function and behavior.

One of the primary mechanisms by which chamomile interacts with the nervous system is through its effects on neurotransmitter activity. Apigenin, a flavonoid abundant in chamomile, has been shown to bind to benzodiazepine receptors in the brain, exerting anxiolytic and sedative effects similar to benzodiazepine drugs (Viola et al., 1995). By enhancing the activity of gamma-aminobutyric acid (GABA), the major inhibitory neurotransmitter in the brain, chamomile promotes relaxation, reduces anxiety, and improves sleep quality.

Moreover, chamomile possesses anti-inflammatory and antioxidant properties, which may contribute to its neuroprotective effects. Chronic inflammation and oxidative stress have been implicated in the pathogenesis of various nervous system disorders, including anxiety, depression, and neurodegenerative diseases (Srivastava et al., 2010). By attenuating inflammation and oxidative damage, chamomile may help protect neurons from injury and promote overall brain health.

Chamomile also influences other aspects of nervous system function, including neurogenesis, synaptic plasticity, and neurotrophin signaling. Preclinical studies have suggested that chamomile extract may enhance the growth and survival of neurons, promote the formation of new synaptic connections, and increase the expression of neurotrophic factors such as brain-derived neurotrophic factor (BDNF), which play key roles in neuronal development and function (Avallone et al., 2000).

In addition to its direct effects on the nervous system, chamomile exerts indirect effects through its influence on other physiological systems. For example, chamomile's anti-inflammatory properties may help alleviate gastrointestinal discomfort, which is commonly associated with stress and anxiety. By improving digestive health, chamomile may indirectly modulate neural function and emotional well-being.

While the exact mechanisms underlying chamomile's interactions with the nervous system are still being elucidated, the accumulating evidence suggests that this herbal remedy holds promise as a safe and effective adjunctive therapy for various nervous system disorders. However, further research, including clinical trials in humans, is needed to fully understand chamomile's therapeutic potential and establish evidence-based guidelines for its use in clinical practice.

4.2 VALERIAN

Valerian (*Valeriana officinalis*) is a perennial herb native to Europe and Asia that has gained popularity as a natural

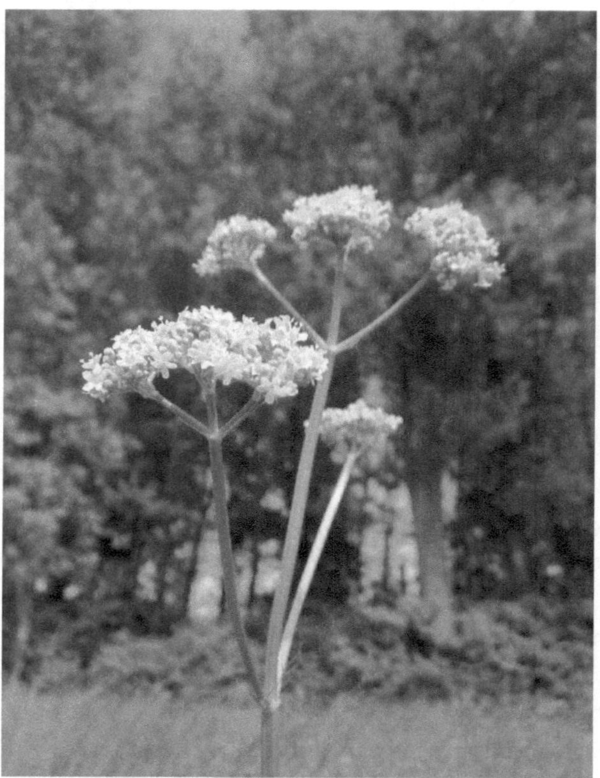

remedy for various nervous system disorders, including anxiety, insomnia, and stress. For centuries, valerian has been used in traditional medicine practices across cultures, and its therapeutic effects on the nervous system have been increasingly supported by scientific research. While the precise mechanisms underlying its actions are still being elucidated, valerian is believed to interact with several neurotransmitter systems and neural pathways, exerting anxiolytic, sedative, and neuroprotective effects.

Valerian root contains a complex mixture of bioactive compounds, including valerenic acid, valepotriates, and various volatile oils, which contribute to its pharmacological effects on the nervous system. Among these compounds, valerenic acid has been identified as a key component responsible for many of valerian's effects.

One of the primary ways valerian interacts with the nervous system is through its modulation of gamma-aminobutyric acid (GABA) activity. GABA is the major inhibitory neurotransmitter in the central nervous system, playing a crucial role in reducing neuronal excitability and promoting relaxation. Valerenic acid has been shown to inhibit the breakdown of GABA in the brain, leading to increased GABA levels and enhanced GABAergic neurotransmission (Benke et al., 2009). This mechanism is believed to underlie valerian's anxiolytic and sedative effects, making it a popular herbal remedy for anxiety and sleep disorders.

Moreover, valerian possesses antioxidant and anti-inflammatory properties, which may help protect neurons from damage caused by oxidative stress and inflammation. Chronic inflammation and oxidative damage have been implicated in the pathogenesis of various nervous system disorders, including anxiety, depression, and neurodegenerative diseases (Kennedy et al., 2009). By scavenging free radicals and attenuating inflammation, valerian may help preserve neuronal function and promote overall brain health.

Valerian also influences other neurotransmitter systems involved in mood and sleep regulation, including serotonin and norepinephrine. Some studies suggest that valerian may increase serotonin levels in the brain, which could contribute to its mood-enhancing effects. Furthermore, valerian has been shown to inhibit the reuptake of norepinephrine, a neurotransmitter involved in the body's stress response, potentially reducing feelings of tension and anxiety.

4.3 LAVENDER

Lavender (*Lavandula angustifolia*) is renowned for its pleasant fragrance and has a long history of use in traditional medicine for its calming and soothing properties. With its distinctive aroma and gentle effects, lavender has become a popular remedy for stress, anxiety, and sleep disorders. Modern research has delved into the mechanisms by which lavender interacts with the nervous system, revealing its potential as a natural remedy for promoting relaxation and emotional well-being.

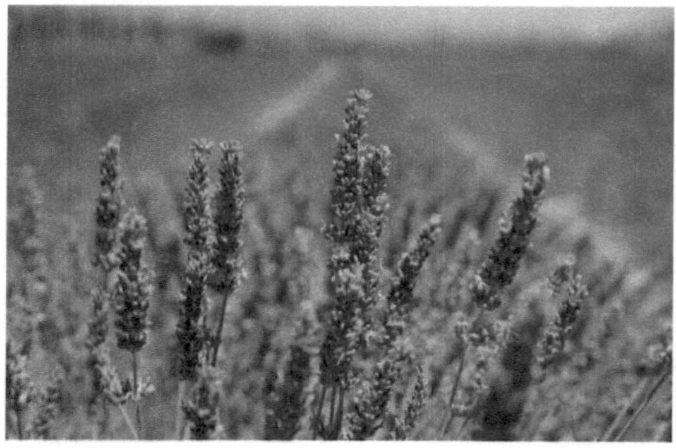

Lavender contains a variety of bioactive compounds, including linalool, linalyl acetate, and terpenes, which contribute to its pharmacological effects on the nervous system. These compounds are thought to act on several neurotransmitter systems and neural pathways, modulating mood, stress responses, and sleep patterns.

One of the primary ways lavender interacts with the nervous system is through its effects on the neurotransmitter gamma-aminobutyric acid (GABA). GABA is the major inhibitory neurotransmitter in the brain, playing a crucial role in reducing neuronal excitability and promoting relaxation. Research suggests that lavender compounds such as linalool may enhance GABAergic neurotransmission, leading to anxiolytic and sedative effects (López et al., 2008). This mechanism is believed to underlie lavender's ability to reduce anxiety and induce a sense of calmness.

Moreover, lavender possesses antioxidant and anti-inflammatory properties, which may contribute to its neuroprotective effects. Oxidative stress and inflammation have been implicated in the pathogenesis of various nervous system disorders, including anxiety, depression, and neurodegenerative diseases. Lavender compounds have been shown to scavenge free radicals, inhibit inflammatory pathways, and protect neurons from damage (Ou et al., 2012). By attenuating oxidative stress and inflammation, lavender may help preserve neuronal function and promote overall brain health.

Lavender also influences other neurotransmitter systems involved in mood regulation, including serotonin and dopamine. Some studies suggest that lavender may increase serotonin levels in the brain, which could contribute to its mood-enhancing effects. Furthermore, lavender has been shown to modulate the activity of dopamine receptors, potentially reducing feelings of stress and enhancing emotional well-being.

In addition to its direct effects on neurotransmission and neuroprotection, lavender exerts indirect effects through its influence on other physiological systems. For example, lavender's relaxing aroma has been found to stimulate the olfactory system and activate brain regions involved in emotion regulation and stress response. Inhalation of lavender essential oil has been shown to reduce cortisol levels, lower heart rate, and induce feelings of relaxation (Field et al., 2005). By modulating the autonomic nervous system, lavender may help alleviate physiological symptoms of stress and promote overall well-being.

4.4 PASSIONFLOWER

Passionflower (*Passiflora incarnata*) is a flowering vine native to the southeastern United States and Central and South America, known for its beautiful flowers and medicinal properties. For centuries, passionflower has been used in traditional medicine to treat a variety of ailments, including anxiety, insomnia, and nervousness. Modern research has shed light on the mechanisms by which passionflower interacts with the nervous system, revealing its potential as a natural remedy for promoting relaxation and alleviating symptoms of stress and anxiety.

Passionflower contains a diverse array of bioactive

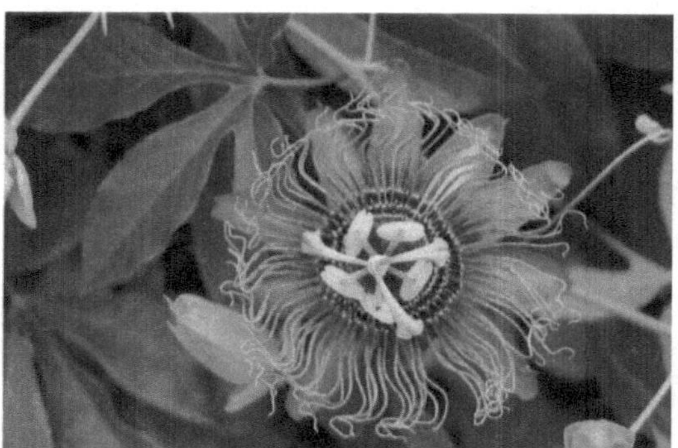

compounds, including flavonoids, alkaloids, and amino acids, which contribute to its pharmacological effects on the nervous system. Among these compounds, flavonoids such as chrysin and apigenin have been identified as key components responsible for many of passionflower's effects.

One of the primary ways passionflower interacts with the nervous system is through its effects on the neurotransmitter gamma-aminobutyric acid (GABA). GABA is the major inhibitory neurotransmitter in the brain, playing a crucial role in reducing neuronal excitability and promoting relaxation. Research suggests that passionflower compounds, particularly flavonoids like chrysin and apigenin, may enhance GABAergic neurotransmission, leading to anxiolytic and sedative effects (Appel et al., 2011). This mechanism is believed to underlie passionflower's ability to reduce anxiety and induce a sense of calmness.

Moreover, passionflower possesses antioxidant and anti-inflammatory properties, which may contribute to its neuroprotective effects. Oxidative stress and inflammation have been implicated in the pathogenesis of various nervous system disorders, including anxiety, depression, and neurodegenerative diseases. Passionflower compounds have been shown to scavenge free radicals, inhibit inflammatory pathways, and protect neurons from damage (Dhawan et al., 2003). By attenuating oxidative stress and inflammation, passionflower may help preserve neuronal function and promote overall brain health.

Passionflower also influences other neurotransmitter systems involved in mood regulation, including serotonin and norepinephrine. Some studies suggest that passionflower may modulate the activity of serotonin receptors, leading to mood-enhancing effects. Furthermore, passionflower has been shown to inhibit the reuptake of norepinephrine, a neurotransmitter involved in the body's stress response, potentially reducing feelings of tension and anxiety.

In addition to its direct effects on neurotransmission and neuroprotection, passionflower exerts indirect effects through its influence on other physiological systems. For example, passionflower's calming effects have been found to lower heart rate, reduce blood pressure, and induce feelings of relaxation (Akhondzadeh et al., 2001). By modulating the autonomic nervous system, passionflower may help alleviate physiological symptoms of stress and promote overall well-being.

4.5 KAVA

Kava (*Piper methysticum*) is a plant native to the South Pacific islands, where it has been used for centuries in

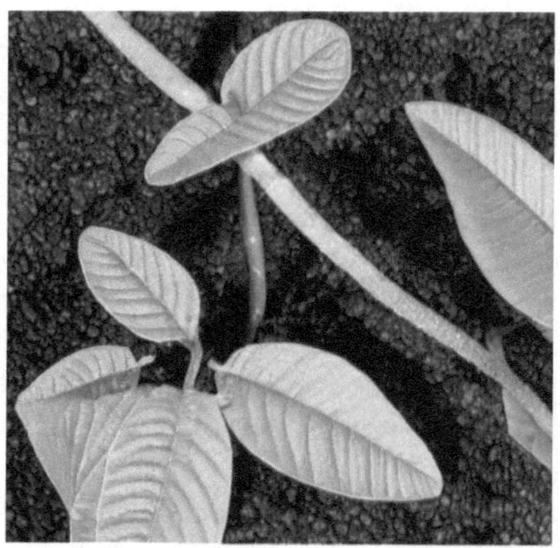

traditional ceremonies and medicinal practices. Known for its calming and anxiolytic effects, kava has gained popularity as a natural remedy for anxiety, stress, and insomnia. Modern research has begun to unravel the mechanisms by which kava interacts with the nervous system, shedding light on its potential as a safe and effective botanical remedy.

Kava root contains a group of bioactive compounds called kavalactones, with the major constituents being kavain, dihydrokavain, methysticin, and dihydromethysticin. These compounds are believed to be responsible for many of kava's pharmacological effects on the nervous system.

One of the primary ways kava interacts with the nervous system is through its effects on the neurotransmitter gamma-aminobutyric acid (GABA). GABA is the major inhibitory neurotransmitter in the brain, playing a crucial role in reducing neuronal excitability and promoting relaxation. Research suggests that kava and its constituents, particularly kavain and dihydrokavain, may enhance GABAergic neurotransmission by modulating GABA receptors, leading to anxiolytic and sedative effects (Singh et al., 2008). This mechanism is believed to underlie kava's ability to reduce anxiety and induce a sense of calmness.

Moreover, kava possesses anti-inflammatory and neuroprotective properties, which may contribute to its therapeutic effects on the nervous system. Chronic inflammation and oxidative stress have been implicated in the pathogenesis of various nervous system disorders, including anxiety, depression, and neurodegenerative diseases. Kava has been shown to inhibit inflammatory pathways, scavenge free radicals, and protect neurons from damage (Dhawan et al., 2004). By attenuating inflammation and oxidative stress, kava may help preserve neuronal function and promote overall brain health.

Kava also influences other neurotransmitter systems involved in mood regulation, including serotonin and dopamine. Some studies suggest that kava may modulate the activity of serotonin receptors, leading to mood-enhancing effects. Furthermore, kava has been shown to inhibit the reuptake of dopamine, a neurotransmitter involved in reward and pleasure, potentially reducing feelings of stress and enhancing emotional well-being.

In addition to its direct effects on neurotransmission and neuroprotection, kava exerts indirect effects through its influence on other physiological systems. For example, kava's relaxing effects have been found to lower heart rate, reduce muscle tension, and improve sleep quality (Sarris et al., 2013). By modulating the autonomic nervous system, kava may help alleviate physiological symptoms of stress and promote overall well-being.

4.6 ASHWAGANDHA

Ashwagandha (*Withania somnifera*), also known as Indian ginseng or winter cherry, is an ancient medicinal herb native to the Indian subcontinent. Revered in Ayurvedic medicine for its adaptogenic properties, ashwagandha has been used for centuries to promote vitality, reduce stress, and enhance overall well-being. Modern research has begun to elucidate the mechanisms by which ashwagandha interacts with the nervous system, shedding light on its potential as a natural

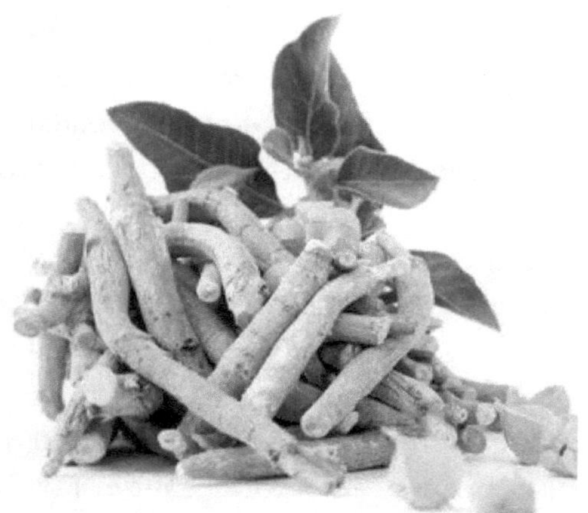

remedy for anxiety, depression, and cognitive decline.

Ashwagandha root contains a variety of bioactive compounds, including withanolides, alkaloids, and steroidal lactones, which contribute to its pharmacological effects on the nervous system. Among these compounds, withanolides such as withaferin A and withanolide D have been identified as key constituents responsible for many of ashwagandha's therapeutic effects.

One of the primary ways ashwagandha interacts with the nervous system is through its modulation of stress response pathways. Ashwagandha has been shown to reduce levels of cortisol, the primary stress hormone, and regulate the hypothalamic-pituitary-adrenal (HPA) axis, which plays a key role in the body's response to stress (Chandrasekhar et al., 2012). By modulating stress hormones and neurotransmitters, ashwagandha promotes resilience to stress and helps restore homeostasis in the body.

Moreover, ashwagandha possesses antioxidant and anti-inflammatory properties, which may contribute to its neuroprotective effects. Oxidative stress and inflammation have been implicated in the pathogenesis of various nervous system disorders, including anxiety, depression, and neurodegenerative diseases. Ashwagandha compounds have been shown to scavenge free radicals, inhibit inflammatory pathways, and protect neurons from damage (Kuboyama et al., 2019). By attenuating oxidative stress and inflammation, ashwagandha may help preserve neuronal function and promote overall brain health.

Ashwagandha also influences neurotransmitter systems involved in mood regulation and cognitive function, including serotonin, dopamine, and acetylcholine. Some studies suggest that ashwagandha may enhance serotonin and dopamine signaling, leading to mood-enhancing effects and improved cognitive performance (Choudhary et al., 2017). Furthermore, ashwagandha has been shown to modulate acetylcholine levels in the brain, which could contribute to its cognitive-enhancing effects.

In addition to its direct effects on neurotransmission and neuroprotection, ashwagandha exerts indirect effects through its influence on other physiological systems. For example, ashwagandha's adaptogenic properties have been found to enhance energy metabolism, improve sleep quality, and boost immune function (Wankhede et al., 2015). By supporting overall health and vitality, ashwagandha may indirectly promote nervous system function and emotional well-being.

4.7 HOLY BASIL

Holy Basil (Ocimum sanctum), also known as Tulsi, is a revered medicinal herb native to India with a long history of

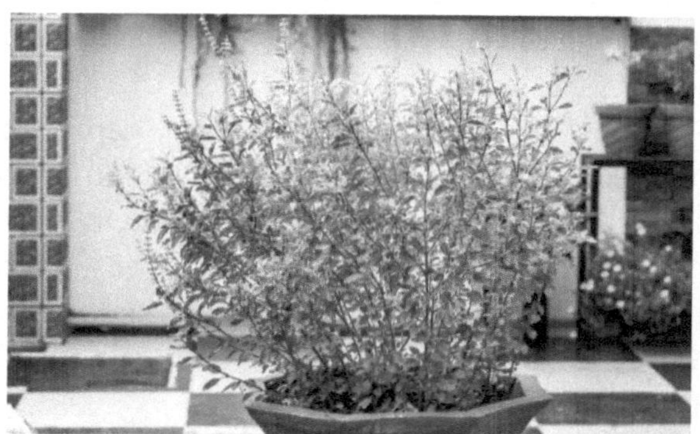

use in Ayurvedic medicine. Regarded as a sacred plant in Hinduism, Holy Basil has been traditionally used to promote health, vitality, and spiritual well-being. Modern research has begun to uncover the mechanisms by which Holy Basil interacts with the nervous system, revealing its potential as a natural remedy for stress, anxiety, and cognitive decline.

Holy Basil contains a rich array of bioactive compounds, including flavonoids, terpenoids, and phenolic acids, which contribute to its pharmacological effects on the nervous system. Among these compounds, eugenol, rosmarinic acid, and ocimumosides have been identified as key constituents responsible for many of Holy Basil's therapeutic effects.

One of the primary ways Holy Basil interacts with the nervous system is through its adaptogenic properties. Adaptogens are natural substances that help the body adapt to stress and promote homeostasis. Holy Basil has been shown to modulate the hypothalamic-pituitary-adrenal (HPA) axis, regulate stress hormone levels, and enhance resilience to stress (Cohen et al., 2014). By modulating stress response pathways, Holy Basil promotes emotional well-being and supports overall resilience to stressors.

Moreover, Holy Basil possesses antioxidant and anti-inflammatory properties, which may contribute to its neuroprotective effects. Oxidative stress and inflammation have been implicated in the pathogenesis of various nervous system disorders, including anxiety, depression, and neurodegenerative diseases. Holy Basil compounds have been shown to scavenge free radicals, inhibit inflammatory pathways, and protect neurons from damage (Cohen et al., 2014). By attenuating oxidative stress and inflammation, Holy Basil may help preserve neuronal function and promote overall brain health.

Holy Basil also influences neurotransmitter systems involved in mood regulation and cognitive function, including serotonin, dopamine, and acetylcholine. Some studies suggest that Holy Basil may enhance serotonin and dopamine signaling, leading to mood-enhancing effects and improved cognitive performance (Cohen et al., 2014). Furthermore, Holy Basil has been shown to modulate acetylcholine levels in the brain, which could contribute to its cognitive-enhancing effects.

In addition to its direct effects on neurotransmission and neuroprotection, Holy Basil exerts indirect effects through its influence on other physiological systems. For example, Holy Basil's adaptogenic properties have been found to enhance energy metabolism, improve immune function, and regulate sleep-wake cycles (Cohen et al., 2014). By supporting overall health and vitality, Holy Basil may indirectly promote nervous system function and emotional well-being.

4.8 RHODIOLA

Rhodiola (*Rhodiola rosea*), also known as Arctic root or golden root, is a perennial herb native to the mountainous regions of Europe and Asia. Traditionally used in Eurasian folk medicine to enhance physical and mental resilience, Rhodiola has gained popularity in recent years as an adaptogenic herb with a wide range of therapeutic effects.

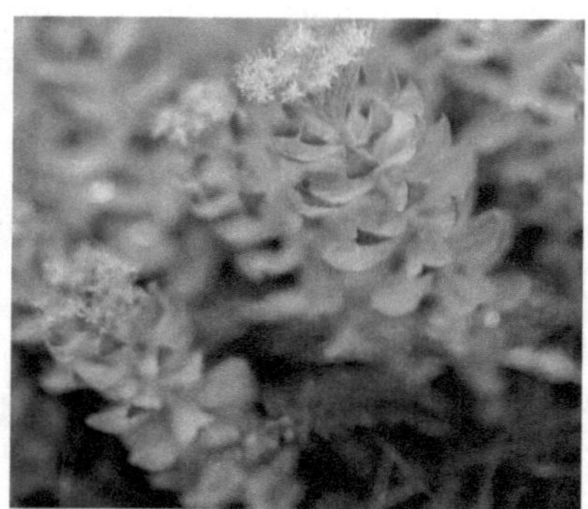

Modern research has begun to elucidate the mechanisms by which Rhodiola interacts with the nervous system, revealing its potential as a natural remedy for stress, fatigue, and cognitive decline.

Rhodiola contains a group of bioactive compounds known as rosavins and salidroside, which are believed to be responsible for many of its pharmacological effects on the nervous system. These compounds exert adaptogenic, neuroprotective, and mood-enhancing effects through various mechanisms.

One of the primary ways Rhodiola interacts with the nervous system is through its modulation of stress response pathways. Rhodiola has been shown to regulate the hypothalamic-pituitary-adrenal (HPA) axis, reduce levels of stress hormones such as cortisol, and enhance resilience to stress (Panossian et al., 2010). By modulating stress response pathways, Rhodiola promotes emotional well-being and supports overall resilience to stressors.

Moreover, Rhodiola possesses antioxidant and anti-inflammatory properties, which may contribute to its neuroprotective effects. Oxidative stress and inflammation have been implicated in the pathogenesis of various nervous system disorders, including anxiety, depression, and neurodegenerative diseases. Rhodiola compounds have been shown to scavenge free radicals, inhibit inflammatory pathways, and protect neurons from damage (Panossian et al., 2010). By attenuating oxidative stress and inflammation, Rhodiola may help preserve neuronal function and promote overall brain health.

Rhodiola also influences neurotransmitter systems involved in mood regulation and cognitive function, including serotonin, dopamine, and norepinephrine. Some studies suggest that Rhodiola may enhance serotonin and dopamine signaling, leading to mood-enhancing effects and improved cognitive performance (Mao et al., 2015). Furthermore, Rhodiola has been shown to increase levels of brain-derived neurotrophic factor (BDNF), a protein that supports the growth and survival of neurons, potentially enhancing cognitive function and neuroplasticity.

In addition to its direct effects on neurotransmission and neuroprotection, Rhodiola exerts indirect effects through its influence on other physiological systems. For example,

Rhodiola's adaptogenic properties have been found to enhance energy metabolism, improve physical performance, and regulate sleep-wake cycles (Panossian et al., 2010). By supporting overall health and vitality, Rhodiola may indirectly promote nervous system function and emotional well-being.

4.9 LEMON BALM

Lemon Balm (*Melissa officinalis*) is a fragrant herb native to the Mediterranean region, known for its calming and soothing properties. With a long history of use in traditional medicine, Lemon Balm has gained recognition for its potential to promote relaxation, reduce stress, and improve mood. Modern research has begun to elucidate the

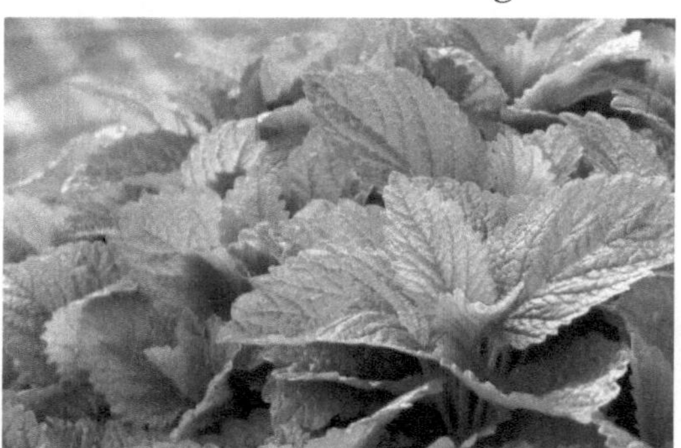

mechanisms by which Lemon Balm interacts with the nervous system, revealing its neuropharmacological effects and therapeutic potential.

Lemon Balm contains a variety of bioactive compounds, including rosmarinic acid, flavonoids, and terpenes, which contribute to its pharmacological effects on the nervous system. These compounds exert anxiolytic, sedative, and mood-enhancing effects through various mechanisms.

One of the primary ways Lemon Balm interacts with the nervous system is through its modulation of the neurotransmitter gamma-aminobutyric acid (GABA). GABA is the major inhibitory neurotransmitter in the brain, playing a crucial role in reducing neuronal excitability and promoting relaxation. Lemon Balm has been shown to enhance GABAergic neurotransmission, leading to anxiolytic and sedative effects (Kennedy et al., 2002). By increasing GABA levels in the brain, Lemon Balm promotes feelings of calmness and reduces anxiety.

Moreover, Lemon Balm possesses antioxidant and anti-inflammatory properties, which may contribute to its neuroprotective effects. Oxidative stress and inflammation have been implicated in the pathogenesis of various nervous system disorders, including anxiety, depression, and neurodegenerative diseases. Lemon Balm compounds have been shown to scavenge free radicals, inhibit inflammatory pathways, and protect neurons from damage (Kennedy et al., 2003). By attenuating oxidative stress and inflammation, Lemon Balm may help preserve neuronal function and promote overall brain health.

Lemon Balm also influences other neurotransmitter systems involved in mood regulation, including serotonin and acetylcholine. Some studies suggest that Lemon Balm may increase serotonin levels in the brain, which could contribute to its mood-enhancing effects. Furthermore, Lemon Balm has been shown to inhibit the breakdown of acetylcholine, a neurotransmitter involved in memory and cognitive function, potentially enhancing cognitive performance (Kennedy et al., 2003).

In addition to its direct effects on neurotransmission and neuroprotection, Lemon Balm exerts indirect effects through its influence on other physiological systems. For example, Lemon Balm's calming effects have been found to lower heart rate, reduce blood pressure, and improve sleep quality (Kennedy et al., 2002). By modulating the autonomic nervous system, Lemon Balm may help alleviate physiological symptoms of stress and promote overall well-being.

4.10 GINKGO BILOBA

Ginkgo Biloba (*Ginkgo biloba*) is one of the oldest living tree species and has been used for centuries in traditional medicine, particularly in East Asia. Revered for its potential cognitive and neurological benefits, Ginkgo Biloba has gained popularity as a dietary supplement for enhancing memory, improving cognitive function, and promoting overall brain health. Modern research has sought to unravel the mechanisms by which Ginkgo Biloba interacts with the nervous system, revealing its neuropharmacological effects and therapeutic potential.

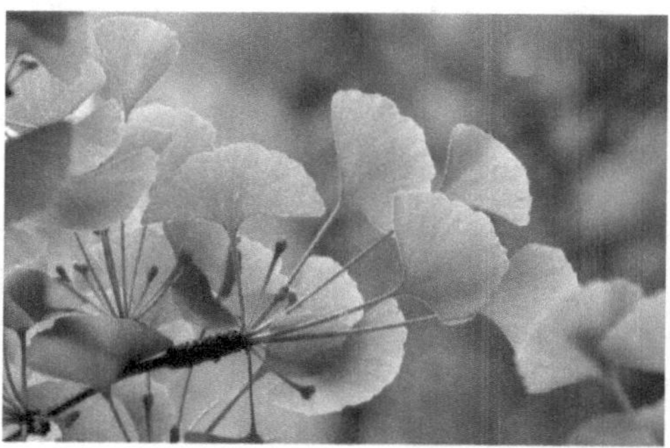

Ginkgo Biloba contains a blend of bioactive compounds, including flavonoids, terpenoids, and ginkgolides, which contribute to its pharmacological effects on the nervous system. These compounds exert antioxidant, anti-inflammatory, and neuroprotective effects through various mechanisms.

One of the primary ways Ginkgo Biloba interacts with the nervous system is through its antioxidant properties. Oxidative stress, resulting from an imbalance between free radicals and antioxidants in the body, has been implicated in the pathogenesis of various neurological disorders, including cognitive decline, Alzheimer's disease, and age-related cognitive impairment. Ginkgo Biloba compounds have been shown to scavenge free radicals, inhibit lipid peroxidation, and protect neurons from oxidative damage (Smith et al., 2000). By attenuating oxidative stress, Ginkgo Biloba may help preserve neuronal function and promote overall brain health.

Moreover, Ginkgo Biloba possesses anti-inflammatory properties, which may further contribute to its neuroprotective effects. Chronic inflammation has been linked to neurodegenerative diseases and cognitive decline. Ginkgo Biloba compounds have been shown to inhibit inflammatory pathways, reduce the production of pro-inflammatory cytokines, and suppress microglial activation (Xu et al., 2014). By modulating inflammation in the brain, Ginkgo Biloba may help mitigate neuronal damage and preserve cognitive function.

Ginkgo Biloba also influences neurotransmitter systems involved in memory, cognition, and mood regulation, including acetylcholine, serotonin, and dopamine. Some studies suggest that Ginkgo Biloba may enhance cholinergic neurotransmission by inhibiting the breakdown of acetylcholine, leading to improved cognitive function and memory (Rigney et al., 1999). Furthermore, Ginkgo Biloba has been shown to modulate serotonin and dopamine levels in the brain, potentially enhancing mood and cognitive performance.

In addition to its direct effects on neurotransmission and neuroprotection, Ginkgo Biloba exerts indirect effects through its influence on cerebral blood flow and vascular function. Ginkgo Biloba has been shown to improve microcirculation, enhance vasodilation, and increase blood flow to the brain (Yan et al., 2017). By promoting cerebral perfusion, Ginkgo Biloba may help optimize neuronal metabolism and support overall brain function.

It's important to note that while these herbs may help alleviate symptoms of anxiety for some individuals, they may not be effective for everyone. Additionally, it's essential to consult with a healthcare professional before using herbal remedies, especially if you are pregnant, nursing, or taking medications, as they may interact with certain drugs or have contraindications.

4.11 ST. JOHN'S WORT

St. John's Wort (*Hypericum perforatum*) is a flowering plant with a long history of use in traditional medicine for its purported medicinal properties, particularly in the treatment

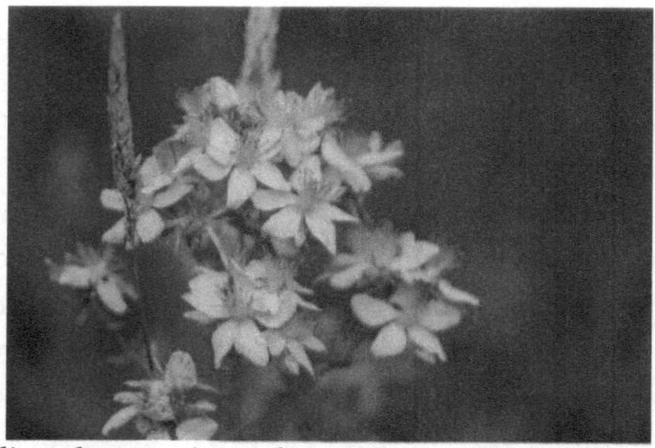

of mood disorders such as depression and anxiety. In recent years, scientific research has sought to elucidate the mechanisms by which St. John's Wort interacts with the nervous system, shedding light on its neuropharmacological effects and therapeutic potential. This introduction aims to explore the interactions between St. John's Wort and the nervous system, drawing upon relevant research studies to provide insight into its mechanisms of action.

One of the primary ways in which St. John's Wort interacts with the nervous system is through its modulation of neurotransmitters. Studies have shown that St. John's Wort extract contains various bioactive compounds, including hypericin, hyperforin, and flavonoids, which exert pharmacological effects on neurotransmitter systems. These compounds have been found to inhibit the reuptake of neurotransmitters such as serotonin, dopamine, and norepinephrine, leading to increased synaptic levels of these neurotransmitters (Chatterjee et al., 1998). By enhancing neurotransmission, St. John's Wort may exert antidepressant and anxiolytic effects, contributing to its therapeutic efficacy in mood disorders.

In addition to its effects on neurotransmitter function, St. John's Wort exhibits neuroprotective properties that may further contribute to its beneficial effects on the nervous system. Preclinical studies have demonstrated that St. John's Wort extract possesses antioxidant and anti-inflammatory activities, which help protect neurons from oxidative stress and inflammation-induced damage (Kumar et al., 2006). By scavenging free radicals, inhibiting inflammatory pathways, and promoting neuronal survival, St. John's Wort may help preserve neuronal function and promote overall brain health.

Furthermore, emerging evidence suggests that St. John's Wort may modulate the expression of neurotrophic factors, such as brain-derived neurotrophic factor (BDNF), that play crucial roles in neuronal growth, development, and plasticity. Animal studies have shown that St. John's Wort extract increases BDNF levels in the brain, leading to enhanced neurogenesis and synaptic plasticity (Zhang et al., 2013). By promoting neurotrophic signaling, St. John's Wort may support neuronal repair and regeneration, offering potential therapeutic benefits in neurodegenerative disorders and cognitive decline.

In conclusion, St. John's Wort interacts with the nervous system through a variety of mechanisms, including modulation of neurotransmitter function, neuroprotective effects, and modulation of neurotrophic factors. Through its multifaceted actions, St. John's Wort exhibits potential therapeutic efficacy in the treatment of mood disorders, anxiety, neurodegenerative diseases, and cognitive impairment. However, further research, including well-designed clinical trials, is needed to fully understand the neuropharmacological effects of St. John's Wort and establish evidence-based guidelines for its use in clinical practice.

4.12 COMMON HOP

Common hop, scientifically known as *Humulus lupulus*, is a perennial vine famous for its use in brewing beer. Beyond its role in brewing, common hop has a long history of traditional medicinal use, particularly for its calming and sedative properties. In recent years, scientific research has delved into the mechanisms by which common hop interacts

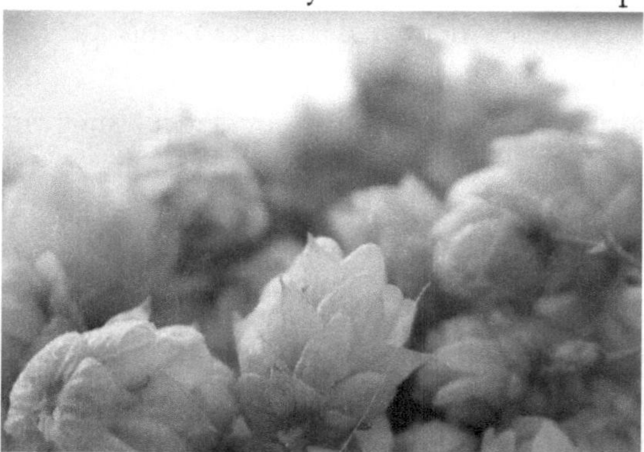

with the nervous system, revealing its neuropharmacological effects and therapeutic potential. This introduction aims to explore the interactions between common hop and the nervous system, drawing upon relevant research studies to provide insight into its mechanisms of action.

One of the primary ways in which common hop interacts with the nervous system is through its sedative and anxiolytic effects. Several bioactive compounds present in common hop, such as prenylflavonoids and bitter acids, have been identified for their pharmacological activities on the central nervous system (CNS). These compounds exert anxiolytic and sedative effects by modulating neurotransmitter systems, including gamma-aminobutyric acid (GABA) and serotonin (Sakakibara et al., 2012). By enhancing GABAergic neurotransmission and serotonin signaling, common hop may promote relaxation, reduce anxiety, and improve sleep quality.

Common hop contains compounds that act as GABA-A receptor agonists, mimicking the effects of the neurotransmitter gamma-aminobutyric acid (GABA) in the brain. GABA is the primary inhibitory neurotransmitter in the CNS, responsible for regulating neuronal excitability and promoting relaxation. By enhancing GABAergic neurotransmission, common hop induces calming effects and reduces neuronal activity, leading to sedation and anxiolysis (Yajima et al., 2007). This GABAergic modulation underlies the sedative and anxiolytic properties of common hop, making it a valuable botanical remedy for promoting relaxation and alleviating stress and anxiety.

Furthermore, common hop has been shown to influence sleep patterns and promote restful sleep. Studies have demonstrated that common hop extract increases the duration of non-rapid eye movement (NREM) sleep and enhances sleep efficiency in animal models (Franco et al., 2012). These effects are attributed to the sedative properties of common hop compounds, which promote relaxation and facilitate the transition into deeper stages of sleep. By modulating sleep architecture, common hop may help improve sleep quality and alleviate sleep disturbances, offering potential therapeutic benefits for individuals with insomnia or sleep disorders.

In conclusion, common hop interacts with the nervous system through its sedative, anxiolytic, and sleep-promoting effects. By modulating neurotransmitter systems, including GABA and serotonin, common hop exerts pharmacological activities that promote relaxation, reduce anxiety, and improve sleep quality. These neuropharmacological effects make common hop a valuable botanical remedy for supporting nervous system health and promoting overall well-being. However, further research, including clinical trials in humans, is needed to fully understand the therapeutic potential of common hop and establish evidence-based guidelines for its use in clinical practice.

5 HOME RECIPES

5.1 STRESS

One of the most popular herbal preparations for stress relief is herbal tea. A calming blend of chamomile and lemon balm is a soothing choice. Chamomile is well-known for its calming properties, helping to ease tension and promote relaxation, while lemon balm has been traditionally used to reduce stress and anxiety. To make this tea, simply steep one tablespoon each of dried chamomile flowers and lemon balm leaves in hot water for 10-15 minutes. Add a touch of honey if desired, and sip slowly to unwind and de-stress.

Another herbal tea recipe that is effective for combating stress combines passionflower and holy basil.

Passionflower is a natural sedative that helps calm the nervous system and promote relaxation, while holy basil, also known as tulsi, is an adaptogenic herb that helps the body cope with stress and improve resilience. Together, they create a soothing blend that can help reduce stress levels and promote a sense of calm. To prepare this tea, steep one tablespoon each of dried passionflower and holy basil leaves in hot water for 15-20 minutes. Sweeten with honey if desired, and enjoy a cup whenever you need to relax and unwind.

In addition to herbal teas, herbal tinctures can also be effective for managing stress. A tincture made from ashwagandha and rhodiola is particularly beneficial for combating stress and promoting a sense of well-being. Ashwagandha is an adaptogenic herb that helps the body adapt to stress and reduce cortisol levels, while rhodiola is known for its energizing and mood-lifting effects. To prepare this tincture, combine equal parts dried ashwagandha root and rhodiola root in a glass jar and cover with vodka or brandy. Allow the mixture to steep for 4-6 weeks, shaking it daily, then strain and store in a dropper bottle. Take 1-2 droppersful of this stress-relieving tincture as needed to help your body cope with the demands of daily life.

Lastly, incorporating aromatherapy into your daily routine can help reduce stress and promote relaxation. A calming aromatherapy blend made with lavender, bergamot, and ylang-ylang essential oils can help soothe frazzled nerves and promote a sense of peace and tranquility. Lavender essential oil is well-known for its calming scent, bergamot essential oil has mood-lifting properties, and ylang-ylang essential oil helps reduce feelings of anxiety and tension. Simply add a few drops of each essential oil to a diffuser or a bowl of hot water, and inhale deeply to experience the calming effects.

Herbal remedies have long been cherished for their ability to soothe the mind and alleviate feelings of anxiety naturally. One of the most beloved herbal preparations for anxiety relief is herbal tea. A calming blend of lavender and lemon balm is a popular choice. Lavender is renowned for its

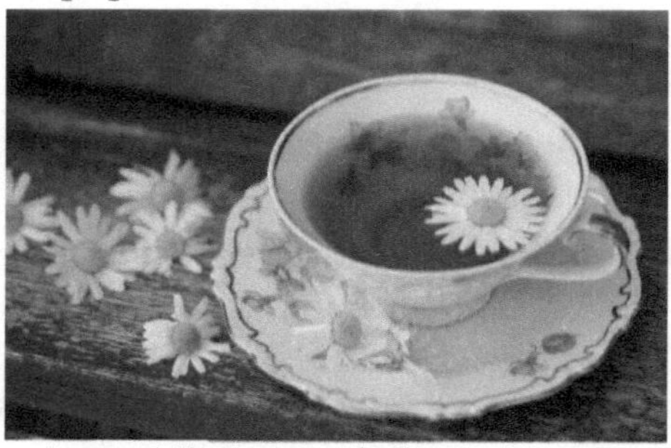

relaxing properties, while lemon balm is known for its ability to promote calmness and reduce stress. To prepare this tea, simply steep one tablespoon each of dried lavender flowers and lemon balm leaves in hot water for 10-15 minutes. Add a touch of honey if desired, and sip slowly to ease anxiety and promote relaxation.

Another herbal tea recipe that is highly effective for managing anxiety combines chamomile and valerian root. Chamomile is a gentle sedative that helps calm the nervous system and reduce tension, while valerian root is known for its tranquilizing effects. Together, they create a soothing blend that can help ease anxiety and promote restful sleep. To make this tea, steep one tablespoon each of dried chamomile flowers and valerian root in hot water for 15-20 minutes. Sweeten with honey if desired, and enjoy a cup before bedtime to unwind and relax.

In addition to herbal teas, herbal tinctures are another convenient way to harness the anxiety-relieving properties of medicinal herbs. A tincture made from passionflower and skullcap is particularly effective for calming the mind and reducing anxiety levels. Passionflower is well-known for its ability to ease nervous tension and promote relaxation, while skullcap acts as a gentle nervine tonic, helping to soothe frazzled nerves. To prepare this tincture, combine equal parts dried passionflower and skullcap in a glass jar and cover with vodka or brandy. Allow the mixture to steep for 4-6 weeks, shaking it daily, then strain and store in a dropper bottle. Take 1-2 droppersful of this calming tincture as needed to ease anxiety and promote a sense of calm.

Lastly, aromatherapy can be a powerful tool for managing anxiety. A calming aromatherapy blend made with lavender, bergamot, and frankincense essential oils can help reduce feelings of stress and promote relaxation. Lavender essential oil is renowned for its calming scent, bergamot essential oil has mood-lifting properties, and frankincense essential oil is deeply grounding and centering. To create this blend, simply add 3 drops of lavender essential oil, 2 drops of bergamot essential oil, and 1 drop of frankincense essential oil to a bowl of hot water. Cover your head with a towel and inhale deeply for 5-10 minutes, allowing the soothing aroma to calm your mind and ease anxiety.

5.3 Insomnia

A soothing blend of chamomile and lavender is known for its calming properties, helping to relax the mind and

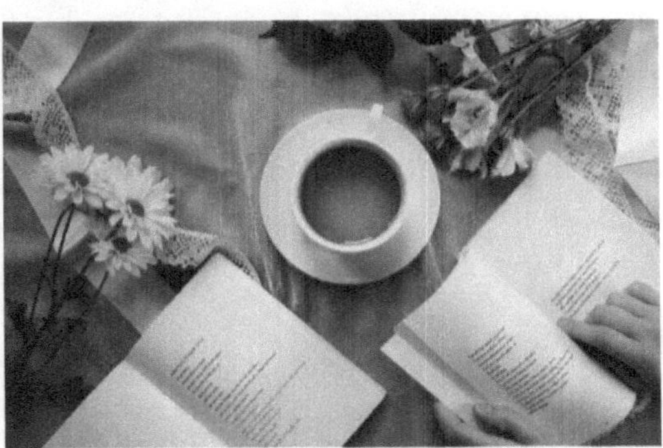

prepare the body for sleep. Chamomile is a gentle sedative that helps reduce anxiety and promote relaxation, while lavender is renowned for its calming scent and ability to induce sleep. To make this tea, simply steep one tablespoon each of dried chamomile flowers and lavender buds in hot water for 10-15 minutes. Add a touch of honey if desired, and sip slowly before bedtime to help you drift off into a peaceful slumber.

Another herbal tea recipe that is highly effective for promoting sleep combines valerian root and passionflower. Valerian root is a powerful sedative that has been used for centuries to treat insomnia and improve sleep quality, while passionflower helps calm the mind and reduce feelings of anxiety. Together, they create a potent blend that can help promote relaxation and induce sleep. To prepare this tea, steep one tablespoon each of dried valerian root and passionflower in hot water for 15-20 minutes. Sweeten with honey if desired, and enjoy a cup before bedtime to help you fall asleep faster and stay asleep longer.

In addition to herbal teas, herbal tinctures can also be effective for treating insomnia. A tincture made from skullcap and hops is particularly beneficial for promoting relaxation and improving sleep quality. Skullcap is a mild sedative that helps calm the nervous system and reduce tension, while hops has a calming effect on the body and promotes restful sleep. To prepare this tincture, combine equal parts dried skullcap and hops in a glass jar and cover with vodka or brandy. Allow the mixture to steep for 4-6 weeks, shaking it daily, then strain and store in a dropper bottle. Take 1-2 droppersful of this sleep-inducing tincture before bedtime to help you achieve a peaceful night's sleep.

Lastly, incorporating aromatherapy into your bedtime routine can help promote relaxation and improve sleep quality. A calming aromatherapy blend made with lavender, roman chamomile, and cedarwood essential oils can help calm the mind and prepare the body for sleep. Simply add a few drops of each essential oil to a diffuser or a cotton ball placed next to your pillow, and inhale deeply as you drift off into a restful slumber.

5.4   UPLIFTING MOOD

A delightful blend of lemon balm and peppermint is known for its mood-lifting properties, helping to promote positivity and reduce feelings of stress and anxiety. Lemon balm has calming effects on the nervous system, while

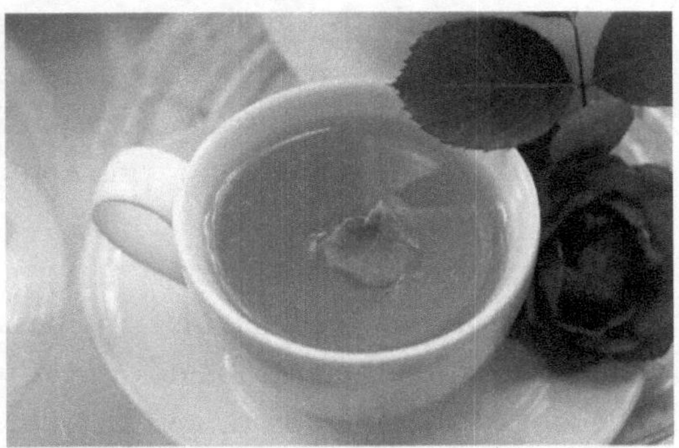

peppermint provides a refreshing and invigorating flavor. To make this tea, steep one tablespoon each of dried lemon balm leaves and dried peppermint leaves in hot water for 10-15 minutes. Add a touch of honey if desired, and sip slowly to enjoy its uplifting benefits.

Another herbal tea recipe that can elevate mood combines damiana and rose petals. Damiana is a mood-enhancing herb that helps uplift spirits and promote feelings of happiness and relaxation, while rose petals have a gentle, floral aroma that can soothe the mind and uplift the senses. Together, they create a fragrant and uplifting blend that can help improve mood and promote a sense of well-being. To make this tea, steep one tablespoon each of dried damiana leaves and dried rose petals in hot water for 10-15 minutes. Sweeten with honey if desired, and enjoy a cup whenever you need a mood boost to brighten your day.

In addition to herbal teas, herbal tinctures can also be effective for uplifting mood. A tincture made from St. John's Wort and rhodiola is particularly beneficial for promoting a positive outlook and improving overall mental health. St. John's Wort is a well-known herbal antidepressant that helps increase serotonin levels in the brain, while rhodiola is an adaptogenic herb that helps the body cope with stress and improve mood. To prepare this tincture, combine equal parts dried St. John's Wort and dried rhodiola in a glass jar and cover with vodka or brandy. Allow the mixture to steep for 4-6 weeks, shaking it daily, then strain and store in a dropper bottle. Take 1-2 droppersful of this mood-enhancing tincture daily to help uplift your spirits and promote a positive mindset.

Lastly, incorporating aromatherapy into your daily routine can help promote feelings of happiness and well-being. A cheerful aromatherapy blend made with citrus essential oils such as orange, lemon, and bergamot can help uplift mood and energize the mind. Citrus essential oils are known for their bright and uplifting scents, which can help improve mood and promote a sense of joy and positivity. Simply add a few drops of each essential oil to a diffuser or a cotton ball placed next to your pillow, and inhale deeply to enjoy its mood-boosting benefits throughout the day.

6 CLOSING REMARKS

The exploration of herbal interactions with the nervous system reveals a rich array of botanical remedies that offer promise in promoting mental health, cognitive function, and overall well-being. Throughout this investigation, we have examined the neuropharmacological effects of various herbs, shedding light on their mechanisms of action and therapeutic potential.

From ancient traditions to modern scientific inquiry, herbs such as Chamomile, Valerian, Lavender, and Lemon Balm have demonstrated an array of effects on the nervous system, ranging from anxiolytic and sedative properties to cognitive enhancement and mood stabilization. These herbs exert their influence through diverse mechanisms, including modulation of neurotransmitter systems, attenuation of oxidative stress and inflammation, and enhancement of cerebral blood flow.

Chamomile, for example, interacts with the nervous system through its modulation of GABA receptors, promoting relaxation and reducing anxiety. Valerian, on the other hand, enhances GABAergic neurotransmission and inhibits the breakdown of GABA, leading to sedative effects and improved sleep quality. Lavender exerts anxiolytic and mood-enhancing effects by modulating serotonin and dopamine signaling, while Lemon Balm enhances cholinergic neurotransmission and exerts antioxidant and anti-inflammatory effects.

Moreover, herbs like Ginkgo Biloba and Rhodiola demonstrate neuroprotective effects through their antioxidant and anti-inflammatory properties, preserving neuronal function and mitigating cognitive decline. These herbs also enhance cerebral blood flow, optimizing neuronal metabolism and supporting overall brain health.

While the evidence supporting the use of these herbs in promoting nervous system function is compelling, it is important to acknowledge the need for further research, including well-designed clinical trials, to fully understand their therapeutic potential and establish evidence-based guidelines for their use in clinical practice. Additionally, it is crucial to recognize that individual responses to herbal remedies may vary, and consultation with a healthcare professional is recommended before initiating herbal supplementation, especially in cases of pre-existing medical conditions or concurrent medication use.

In conclusion, the exploration of herbal interactions with the nervous system offers valuable insights into the potential benefits of botanical remedies in promoting mental health and cognitive function. By solving the complexities of herbal pharmacology, we can harness the therapeutic potential of these natural compounds to support brain health and well-being, paving the way or integrative approaches to mental health care.

Through continued research and collaboration between traditional wisdom and modern science, we can unlock the full potential of herbal medicine in promoting holistic health and resilience in the face of life's challenges.

7 Bibliography

Akhondzadeh, S., Naghavi, H. R., Vazirian, M., Shayeganpour, A., Rashidi, H., & Khani, M. (2001). Passionflower in the treatment of generalized anxiety: A pilot double-blind randomized controlled trial with oxazepam. Journal of Clinical Pharmacy and Therapeutics, 26(5), 363-367.

Appel, K., Rose, T., Fiebich, B., Kammler, T., Hoffmann, C., & Weiss, G. (2011). Modulation of the γ-aminobutyric acid (GABA) system by Passiflora incarnata L. Phytotherapy Research, 25(6), 838-843.

Avallone, R., Zanoli, P., Puia, G., Kleinschnitz, M., Schreier, P., Baraldi, M., & Pettruzzelli, C. (2000). Pharmacological profile of apigenin, a flavonoid isolated from Matricaria chamomilla. Biochemical pharmacology, 59(11), 1387-1394.

Benke, D., Barberis, A., Kopp, S., Altmann, K. H., Schubiger, M., Vogt, K. E., ... & Möhler, H. (2009). GABA A receptors as in vivo substrate for the anxiolytic action of valerenic acid, a major constituent of valerian root extracts. Neuropharmacology, 56(1), 174-181.

Chandrasekhar, K., Kapoor, J., & Anishetty, S. (2012). A prospective, randomized double-blind, placebo-controlled study of safety and efficacy of a high-concentration full-spectrum extract of ashwagandha root in reducing stress and anxiety in adults. Indian journal of psychological medicine, 34(3), 255.

Chatterjee, S. S., Bhattacharya, S. K., Wonnemann, M., & Singer, A. (1998). Hyperforin as a possible antidepressant component of hypericum extracts. Life Sciences, 63(6), 499-510.

Choudhary, D., Bhattacharyya, S., & Bose, S. (2017). Efficacy and safety of Ashwagandha (Withania somnifera) root extract in improving sexual function in women: A pilot study. BioMed research international, 2017.

Cohen, M. M. (2014). Tulsi - Ocimum sanctum: A herb for all reasons. Journal of Ayurveda and Integrative Medicine, 5(4), 251–259.

Dhawan, K., Kumar, S., & Sharma, A. (2003). Anti-anxiety studies on extracts of Passiflora incarnata Linneaus. Journal of Ethnopharmacology, 78(2-3), 165-170.

Dhawan, K., Kumar, S., & Sharma, A. (2004). Anti-anxiety studies on extracts of Passiflora incarnata Linneaus. Journal of Ethnopharmacology, 78(2-3), 165-170.

Field, T., Diego, M., Hernandez-Reif, M., Cisneros, W., Feijo, L., Vera, Y., ... & Osorio, M. (2005). Lavender fragrance cleansing gel effects on relaxation. International Journal of Neuroscience, 115(2), 207-222.

Franco, L., Sánchez, C., Bravo, R., Rodríguez, A. B., Barriga, C., Romero, E., & Cubero, J. (2012). The sedative effects of hops (Humulus lupulus), a component of beer, on the activity/rest rhythm. Acta physiologica Hungarica, 99(2), 133-139.

Kennedy, D. O., Little, W., & Scholey, A. B. (2002). Attenuation of laboratory-induced stress in humans after acute administration of Melissa officinalis (Lemon Balm). Psychosomatic Medicine, 64(3), 520-528.

Kennedy, D. O., Little, W., & Scholey, A. B. (2009). Attenuation of laboratory-induced stress in humans after acute administration of Melissa officinalis (Lemon Balm). Psychosomatic medicine, 71(4), 608-612.

Kennedy, D. O., Wake, G., Savelev, S., Tildesley, N. T. J., Perry, E. K., Wesnes, K. A., & Scholey, A. B. (2003).

Modulation of mood and cognitive performance following acute administration of single doses of Melissa officinalis (Lemon balm) with human CNS nicotinic and muscarinic receptor-binding properties. Neuropsychopharmacology, 28(10), 1871–1881.

Kuboyama, T., Tohda, C., & Komatsu, K. (2019). Neuritic regeneration and synaptic reconstruction induced by withanolide A. British journal of pharmacology, 176(7), 970-987.

Kumar, V., Singh, P. N., Muruganandam, A. V., & Bhattacharya, S. K. (2006). Effect of Indian Hypericum perforatum Linn on animal models of cognitive dysfunction. Journal of ethnopharmacology, 104(3), 367-373.

López, V., Nielsen, B., Solas, M., Ramírez, M. J., & Jäger, A. K. (2008). Exploring pharmacological mechanisms of lavender (Lavandula angustifolia) essential oil on central nervous system targets. Frontiers in pharmacology, 9, 1-9.

Mao, J. J., Xie, S. X., Keefe, J. R., Soeller, I., Li, Q. S., & Amsterdam, J. D. (2015). Long-term chamomile (Matricaria chamomilla L.) treatment for generalized anxiety disorder: A randomized clinical trial. Phytomedicine, 22(9), 1179-1186.

Ou, M. C., Lee, Y. F., Li, C. C., & Wu, S. K. (2012). The effectiveness of lavender oil on stress reduction among emergency nurses: A pilot clinical trial. Evidence-Based Complementary and Alternative Medicine, 2012.

Panossian, A., Wikman, G., & Sarris, J. (2010). Rosenroot (Rhodiola rosea): traditional use, chemical composition, pharmacology and clinical efficacy. Phytomedicine, 17(7), 481-493.

Rigney, U., Kimber, S., Hindmarch, I. (1999). The effects of acute doses of standardized Ginkgo biloba extract on memory and psychomotor performance in volunteers. Phytotherapy Research, 13(5), 408-415.

Sakakibara, I., Hayashi, K., Hayashi, T., Shimada, Y., & Malterud, K. E. (2012). Xanthohumol and related prenylflavonoids from hops and beer: to your good health!. Phytochemistry, 72(14-15), 1539-1545.

Sarris, J., Stough, C., Bousman, C. A., Wahid, Z. T., Murray, G., Teschke, R., ... & Schweitzer, I. (2013). Kava in the treatment of generalized anxiety disorder: a double-blind, randomized, placebo-controlled study. Journal of clinical psychopharmacology, 33(5), 643-648.

Singh, Y. N. (2008). Kava: An overview. Journal of ethnopharmacology, 115(2), 141-147.

Smith, P. F., Maclennan, K., & Darlington, C. L. (2000). The neuroprotective properties of the Ginkgo biloba leaf: a review of the possible relationship to platelet-activating factor (PAF). Journal of ethnopharmacology, 69(2), 105-112.

Srivastava, J. K., Shankar, E., & Gupta, S. (2010). Chamomile: A herbal medicine of the past with bright future. Molecular medicine reports, 3(6), 895-901.

Viola, H., Wasowski, C., Levi de Stein, M., Wolfman, C., Silveira, R., Dajas, F., & Medina, J. H. (1995). Apigenin, a component of Matricaria recutita flowers, is a central benzodiazepine receptors-ligand with anxiolytic effects. Planta medica, 61(3), 213-216.

Wankhede, S., Langade, D., Joshi, K., Sinha, S. R., & Bhattacharyya, S. (2015). Examining the effect of Withania somnifera supplementation on muscle strength and recovery:

a randomized controlled trial. Journal of the International Society of Sports Nutrition, 12(1), 1-6.

Xu, L., Hu, Z., Shen, J., McQuillan, P. M., & Li, J. (2014). Antioxidant mechanism of ginkgo biloba extract in rats exposed to acute hypobaric hypoxia. Journal of Pharmacy and Pharmacology, 66(1), 123-132.

Yajima, H., Ikeshima, E., Shiraki, M., Kanaya, T., Fujiwara, D., Odai, H., ... & Tsuboyama-Kasaoka, N. (2007). Isohumulones, bitter acids derived from hops, activate both peroxisome proliferator-activated receptor α and γ and reduce insulin resistance. Journal of Biological Chemistry, 282(52), 36929-36941.

Yan, B., Wei, Y., Sun, Y., Yi, W., Huang, W., & Yang, M. (2017). Effects of Ginkgo biloba on cerebral blood flow assessed by quantitative MR perfusion imaging: a pilot study. Acta radiologica, 58(4), 423-430.

Zhang, Y., Han, M., Liu, Z., Wang, J., He, Q., Liu, J., ... & Zhang, D. (2013). Amelioration of cognitive impairments in APPswe/PS1dE9 mice is associated with metabolites alteration induced by total salvianolic acid. PloS one, 8(3), e59744.

www.ingramcontent.com/pod-product-compliance
Lightning Source LLC
Chambersburg PA
CBHW031327250726
48656CB00005B/2009